Evaluation of Environmental Controls at a Social Assistance Facility (Community Rehabilitation Center) Associated with a Tuberculosis Outbreak – Florida

Stephen B. Martin, Jr., MS, PE
Kenneth R. Mead, PhD, PE
R. Brent Lawrence, MS, GSP
Michael C. Beaty

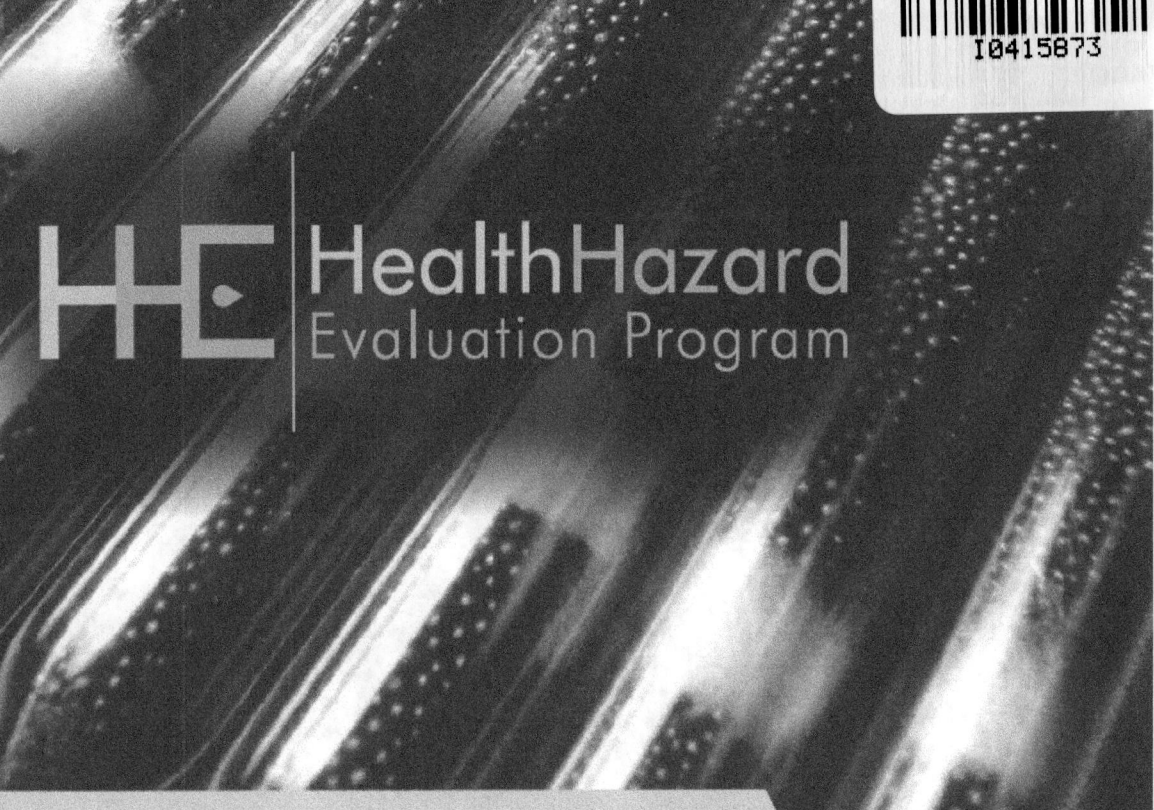

HealthHazard
Evaluation Program

I0415873

Report No. 2012-0263-3181
July 2013

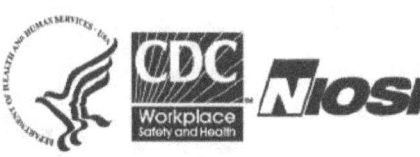

U.S. Department of Health and Human Services
Centers for Disease Control and Prevention
National Institute for Occupational Safety and Health

CDC
Workplace
Safety and Health

NIOSH

Contents

Highlights of this Evaluation

The National Institute for Occupational Safety and Health received a technical assistance request from the Duval County Health Department in Florida. The request asked that we assess the heating, ventilation, and air-conditioning systems and make recommendations to improve overall environmental controls at Community Rehabilitation Center, a local social assistance facility with epidemiological links to an ongoing tuberculosis outbreak.

What NIOSH Did

- We visited Community Rehabilitation Center on August 21, 2012.

- We met with representatives from the Duval County Health Department and Community Rehabilitation Center to discuss the ongoing tuberculosis outbreak.

- We recorded the physical sizes of occupied spaces.

- We measured ventilation air flow into/from all occupied spaces.

- We collected information on facility air-handling units.

What NIOSH Found

- Community Rehabilitation Center was working in conjunction with the Duval County Health Department to improve administrative controls to identify guests on priority screening lists or those with symptoms of tuberculosis.

- Central air-handling units in the main building were in good working order and had proper filter configurations installed.

- Some window ventilation units in the old portion of the main building were not operational.

- No fresh outdoor air was being supplied to the occupied spaces by building mechanical systems.

- A written respiratory protection plan did not exist.

- Most bathroom exhaust fans were not properly maintaining the spaces under negative pressure.

What Community Rehabilitation Center Should Do

- Continue to work with the Duval County Health Department to improve overall administrative controls and help ensure rapid identification of guests suspected to have tuberculosis.

- Develop a comprehensive infection control plan with input from the Duval County Health Department and Florida Department of Health.

- Modify facility ventilation systems to provide adequate fresh outdoor air to all occupied spaces using a strategy compatible with existing system capacities.

- Replace all existing packaged terminal air conditioner units in the old portion of the main building with a new, efficient central air-handling unit.

- Install the highest efficiency air filters possible that is consistent with the proper operation of each air-handling unit.

- Develop and implement a written respiratory protection program that meets the requirements of the Occupational Safety and Health Administration's respiratory protection respiratory protection standard 29 Code of Federal Regulations 1910.134.

- Adjust supply air flow into bathrooms so spaces are maintained under negative pressure during occupancy and repair or replace bathroom exhaust fans not meeting performance specifications.

- Develop and implement a written operation and maintenance plan for all facility heating, ventilation, and air-conditioning systems, to include a filter replacement schedule.

Abbreviations

μm	Micrometer
AHU(s)	Air-handling unit(s)
ANSI®	American National Standards Institute
ASHRAE®	American Society of Heating, Refrigerating and Air-Conditioning Engineers
CDC	Centers for Disease Control and Prevention
cfm	Cubic feet per minute
CFR	Code of Federal Regulations
DCHD	Duval County Health Department
DRDS	Division of Respiratory Disease Studies
DTBE	Division of Tuberculosis Elimination
ft²	Square feet
HVAC	Heating, ventilation, and air-conditioning
ICP	Infection control plan
MERV	Minimum efficiency reporting value
NCHHSTP	National Center for HIV/AIDS, Viral Hepatitis, STD, and TB Prevention
NIOSH	National Institute for Occupational Safety and Health
O&M	Operation and maintenance
OSHA	Occupational Safety and Health Administration
PTAC	Packaged terminal air conditioner
RH	Relative humidity
TB	Tuberculosis

Mention of any company or product does not constitute endorsement by NIOSH. In addition, citations to websites external to NIOSH do not constitute NIOSH endorsement of the sponsoring organizations or their programs or products. Furthermore, NIOSH is not responsible for the content of these websites. All web addresses referenced in this document were accessible as of the publication date of this report.

Summary

In May 2012, the National Institute for Occupational Safety and Health (NIOSH) received a request for technical assistance from the Duval County Health Department as part of its response to an ongoing tuberculosis (TB) outbreak among homeless persons in Florida. The request asked NIOSH to assess heating, ventilation, and air-conditioning (HVAC) systems and make recommendations to improve overall environmental controls at four homeless facilities with epidemiologic links to past or ongoing TB disease transmission.

During an on-site evaluation of the Community Rehabilitation Center social assistance facility in August 2012, we collected physical and ventilation measurements in all key areas of the facility. We focused on areas where guests typically congregate or spend significant amounts of time. We recorded the make and model number of air-handling units (AHUs) providing supply air to the facility, and visually inspected the units. When possible, we measured the air flow rate through supply diffusers and return grilles.

NIOSH investigators conducted an assessment of environmental controls in Community Rehabilitation Center, a social assistance facility linked to an ongoing tuberculosis outbreak. The investigation revealed problems with the existing environmental controls, along with needed improvements in administrative controls and respiratory protection. Detailed recommendations are provided in this report to improve the shelter environment and reduce the likelihood of disease transmission.

The ventilation systems in place could have contributed to airborne disease transmission among facility guests. With the exception of some window units in the older portion of the main building, the AHUs appeared adequately maintained and were fully operational. Unfortunately, none of the AHUs provided fresh outdoor air to the occupied spaces, as required by the *Florida Building Code* and American Society of Heating, Refrigerating and Air-Conditioning Engineers design standards. In addition to alleviating odors and maintaining occupant comfort, outdoor air serves to dilute infectious aerosols, such as *Mycobacterium tuberculosis* droplet nuclei that are responsible for TB transmission.

Since the TB outbreak began, Community Rehabilitation Center has taken numerous steps to improve administrative controls, particularly when it comes to identifying guests showing signs and symptoms of TB. We recommend additional improvements to the administrative and environmental controls at the center. From a ventilation standpoint, we suggest that all occupied spaces in the facility are supplied adequate amounts of outdoor air. We also recommend developing a written infection control plan, HVAC operation and maintenance plan, and a written respiratory protection program. Having these plans/programs in place will help the center under normal operating conditions, and especially during future outbreaks of respiratory disease.

Keywords: NAICS 624310 (Vocational Rehabilitation Services), tuberculosis, environmental controls, ventilation, adult education facility, airborne infection, airborne transmission, respiratory

Introduction

Since 2004, the Duval County Health Department (DCHD), in conjunction with the Florida Department of Health and U.S. Centers for Disease Control and Prevention (CDC), has linked over 100 cases of active tuberculosis (TB) disease, resulting in 14 deaths, to a cluster having matching genotype results (PCR00160 or FL0046) in Duval County, Florida. Roughly half of the cases of active TB disease have been identified since 2010. Of the 100 cases, 79% had a history of homelessness, incarceration, or substance abuse, with 43% being homeless within one year of diagnosis.

In response to the ongoing outbreak, a team of epidemiologists from the CDC National Center for HIV/AIDS, Viral Hepatitis, STD, and TB Prevention (NCHHSTP), Division of Tuberculosis Elimination (DTBE) conducted an on-site investigation in February and March 2012. In their report dated April 5, 2012, the CDC team included a recommendation to improve environmental controls at homeless facilities implicated in possible disease transmission. On May 22, 2012, the Division of Respiratory Disease Studies (DRDS), National Institute for Occupational Safety and Health (NIOSH), CDC received a request for technical assistance concerning the TB outbreak in Duval County. The request was made by a CDC Public Health Advisor temporarily assigned to Duval County. The request specifically asked NIOSH to evaluate shelters' heating, ventilation, and air-conditioning (HVAC) systems and make recommendations to improve overall environmental controls. The request was initially made for an assessment at one homeless shelter. However, in subsequent discussions with the TB Program Manager at DCHD, a CDC Public Health Advisor with the Florida Department of Health, and representatives from CDC/NCHHSTP/DTBE, the request was expanded to include four facilities that provide assistance to the homeless and which had epidemiologic links to past or ongoing TB disease transmission.

In response to the expanded request, a NIOSH team visited the four facilities in August 2012. This report describes the measurements and associated findings from our assessment at Community Rehabilitation Center. It details and prioritizes our recommendations for improving environmental controls at the facility, and outlines the current plan for future NIOSH involvement.

Background

Tuberculosis and Homeless Populations
TB is a disease caused by *Mycobacterium tuberculosis (M. tuberculosis)* bacteria. When a

person with active TB disease coughs or sneezes, tiny droplets containing *M. tuberculosis* may be expelled into the air. Many of these droplets dry, and the resulting residues remain suspended in the air for long periods of time as droplet nuclei. If another person inhales air that contains the infectious droplet nuclei, transmission from one person to another may occur. Homeless people have been identified as a high-risk population for TB infection and disease since the early 1900s [Knopf 1914]. With the increase in homelessness in the United States since the 1980s, TB among homeless persons has become a subject of heightened interest and concern [CDC 1985; 1992; 2003a,b; 2005a; Barry et al. 1986; Slutkin 1986; McAdam et al. 1990; Nolan 1991].

Community Rehabilitation Center

The Community Rehabilitation Center social assistance facility was established in 1993 and is primarily an outpatient mental health facility serving people in Duval and surrounding counties. The facility offers behavioral care, primary care, and community economic development services for individuals at the poverty level with mental illness, substance abuse or HIV/AIDS. It employs more than 60 professionals that work in all service areas provided by the center. Approximately 160 clients come to the facility each day to participate in educational and vocational day programs between 9:00 AM–12:00 PM and/or 2:00 PM–6:00 PM. Transportation to/from the facility is provided for clients that need it. This facility differed from the other three we visited in that it was the only facility that did not house overnight clients.

The main structure is a 16,000 square feet (ft^2), one-story masonry building. The building is divided nearly in half between newer and older portions. The newer portion houses the main entrance and reception areas, two large dining/activity areas that can be opened up to one large space, a kitchen, conference room, and many staff offices. The new portion is equipped with two central heating and air conditioning systems that provide ventilation to all spaces in that section of the facility. The older portion of the structure houses several staff offices, a break room, and seven team rooms. Four team rooms are on one side of a hallway, and three are on the other. Dividers between the team rooms can be opened and closed to combine/separate spaces to house classes of various sizes. Most of the staff offices in the old building are ventilated by one rooftop air-handling unit. However, the team rooms and offices down the longest hallway are ventilated with under-window packaged terminal air conditioner (PTAC) units.

Adjacent to the main building are two trailers used as counseling areas for clients and a small two-story masonry drop-off building. The smaller of the two trailers has an office and adult education area. It is ventilated by a central HVAC unit installed on one end. The larger trailer has two central HVAC units providing ventilation to six offices, a waiting area, and reception space. The drop-off building has a central AHU in the attic that provides ventilation to a large client gathering area on the first floor. Clients use this space before and after scheduled programs and during periods of bad weather.

In 2006, Community Rehabilitation Center expanded their services to include a thrift shop and a screen print shop located near the main building. However, these facilities were not visited as part of our technical assistance response.

Assessment

On August 20, 2012, an opening meeting was held at the Duval County Health Department. An update was given on the current status of the ongoing TB outbreak among the homeless population, and we provided background information on NIOSH, the nature of the technical assistance request, and the ventilation measurements we planned to collect at each facility. Aside from NIOSH and DCHD staff, representatives from Community Rehabilitation Center and two of the three other homeless facilities to be visited were in attendance.

We arrived at Community Rehabilitation Center on Tuesday, August 21, 2012 and signed into the building. After we unloaded our equipment, the facilities manager provided us with floor plans of the main building and led a tour of the entire facility. After the tour, we began taking physical and ventilation measurements in all key areas. We focused on areas where clients typically congregate or spend significant amounts of time, but measurements were taken throughout the entire facility.

We recorded the make and model number of all central AHUs providing supply air to the facility, and we visually inspected the units. When possible, we measured the air flow rate through supply diffusers and return grilles using a TSI Incorporated (Shoreview, Minnesota) Model 8373 Accubalance Plus equipped with an appropriate air capture hood. The Model 8373 measures volumetric air flow rates of 30–2000 cubic feet per minute (cfm) with an accuracy of ±5% of the reading and ±5 cfm. The Accubalance Plus is also equipped with a directional air flow indicator that provides confirmation of flow direction. We determined the approximate internal volume of the measured spaces with either a standard tape measure or a Zircon Corporation (Campbell, California) Model 58026 LaserVision DM200 laser distance measuring device. The device accurately measures up to 200 feet and has function keys for calculating the area and volume of a room for HVAC load formulas. When the existence of air flow or the air flow direction was questioned, we used a Wizard Stick hand-held fog generator (Zero Toys, Concord, Massachusetts) to confirm and visualize the air flow pattern.

After recording our measurements, we met briefly with the Community Rehabilitation Center facilities manager on the afternoon of August 22, 2013 to discuss our general findings from our previous day's assessment. A formal closing meeting for our on-site response to the technical assistance request for all four of the facilities was held on August 23, 2012, at the DCHD. This meeting provided us an opportunity to discuss our general findings with representatives from the Duval County Health Department.

Results and Discussion

General Tuberculosis Infection Control

All tuberculosis control programs should include three key components: administrative controls (e.g., intake questionnaires and policies), environmental controls (e.g., ventilation and filtration), and a respiratory protection program. Ideally, environmental controls and respiratory protection should supplement aggressive administrative controls. Detailed explanations for each of these key control elements, as well as a discussion on the hierarchy of their implementation, are outlined in CDC's *Guidelines for Preventing the Transmission of* Mycobacterium tuberculosis *in Health-Care Settings, 2005 and Prevention and Control of Tuberculosis in Correctional and Detention Facilities: Recommendations from CDC* [CDC 2005b, 2006]. In high risk environments, such as this social assistance facility, or in areas where administrative controls alone are inadequate, environmental controls and respiratory protection should be used as secondary and tertiary levels of control, respectively.

Administrative Controls

During our visit, and in previous conversations with representatives from DTBE, the Florida Department of Health, DCHD, and Community Rehabilitation Center, it was apparent that limited TB administrative controls were in place at the facility prior to the current disease outbreak. However, efforts were taken to improve the overall administrative controls in place at the time of the site visit. Employees were trained on symptoms of TB disease and prevention of TB transmission. Additionally, intake screening procedures are now in place to help identify clients on target screening lists, or others suspected of having TB, and refer them to DCHD for critical medical screening. These procedures will help identify infected individuals more rapidly in the future and serve to help keep infected clients away from those that are healthy.

We cannot overstate the importance of having robust administrative controls in place. The overall mission of the facility typically results in services being provided to large numbers of clients, often in close proximity to one another. This is particularly the case in the dining/assembly areas and the team rooms. Even the best ventilation systems are incapable of preventing the spread of disease between two clients close to one another. Thus, identifying people with suspected disease, keeping them separated from the general client population, and following up with appropriate medical evaluations and treatment (if necessary) are the most important elements of reducing or eliminating the spread of disease.

While enhancing administrative controls is a significant step, the development of a written TB Infection Control Plan (ICP) for the facility should be considered. At the time of the NIOSH investigation, no such ICP was reported to exist. Information on creating detailed ICPs and TB ICP templates can be found at the Curry International Tuberculosis Center website at http://www.currytbcenter.ucsf.edu/. Collaborating with DCHD and the Florida Department of Health would serve to further strengthen the written plan. These ICPs are particularly useful when overall TB infection control requires the coordination and subsequent follow-up of different agencies. In response to this current TB outbreak, there was good communication and coordination between Community Rehabilitation Center and DCHD. However, the process should be formally documented in a protocol or checklist format. This ensures that each time there is a TB-related incident, all necessary agencies understand their responsibilities and perform their necessary predetermined actions in a consistent manner. Incorporating the input of staff involved in the maintenance and operation of facility ventilation systems into the overall infection control program strengthens the program and provides these staff members with additional insight as to what ventilation requirements are necessary to prevent and/or isolate TB disease. Input from the ventilation staff should be sought during the formal creation of the ICP and during subsequent revisions to the plan.

Environmental Controls
<u>General Ventilation System Information</u>
General information on the central AHUs at Community Rehabilitation Center, including the areas served by each unit, is provided in Table 1. All three of the central AHUs supplying air to the main building were fairly new, and on the day of our visit, were fully maintaining temperature set points and air flow. AHU-1 and AHU-2, servicing the newer portion of the building, were installed in a mechanical room adjacent to the Executive Director's office. In addition to housing the two AHUs, the mechanical space was also used for storage. Gaining access to the AHUs was difficult because of the additional clutter in the space, but it was determined that the two AHUs were manufactured in late 2000 or early 2001. AHU-3, a roof-top unit that services part of the older section of the building, was manufactured in June 2012 and installed just prior to our visit. Each of the main building AHUs supply air to occupied spaces through galvanized steel supply ducts. Return air flows back to the units in the new portion of the building through ducted returns. Return air back to AHU-3 is mainly via a ceiling plenum, with air from the occupied spaces traveling to the plenum around light fixtures and through holes in the drop ceiling. All three of these central AHUs had properly-sized filter configurations during our visit. However, none of the units delivered fresh, outdoor air to the occupied spaces. The configuration for AHU-3 had dedicated capacity for introducing outdoor air, but the outdoor air dampers were sealed shut and not operable.

The window PTAC units installed along the longest hallway of the older portion of the main building were from various manufacturers. While most appeared to be functional, some were not in use during our visit. Information on the make/model of each PTAC unit was not recorded since the units were not intended to bring in any fresh, outdoor air and only served to condition and recirculate air within the same space(s) they served.

The AHUs in the two trailers appeared to be installed during the production of the trailers themselves. While the two units servicing the large trailer were produced by Eubank Manufacturing Enterprises (Longview, Texas), an exact date of manufacturing could not be determined. All of the labels and stickers on the single AHU servicing the small trailer were missing or faded to the point they could not be read (see Table 1). These units provided supply air through ductwork installed in the ceiling of each trailer. Return air to the trailer AHUs traveled through grilles in the walls of the individual spaces, into the main hallway of each trailer, and directly back to the AHUs themselves. These AHUs were all equipped with air filters.

We were unable to gain access to the AHU servicing the assembly area/game room in the drop off building. Thus, the make/model, supply and return schemes, and filter configuration could not be determined. This space was completely unoccupied during the NIOSH visit and was only reported to be used for short periods of time before and after classes or during periods of bad weather.

Filtration

All of the ventilation filters used in the main building central AHUs had an American Society of Heating, Refrigerating and Air-Conditioning Engineers (ASHRAE) Minimum Efficiency Reporting Value (MERV) of 8, which corresponds to a removal efficiency of greater than 70% for 3.0 to 10 micrometer (μm) particles [ANSI/ASHRAE 2007]. However, MERV 8 filters are only around 25% efficient at filtering particles in the 1.0–3.0 μm size range, which includes droplet nuclei responsible for *M. tuberculosis* transmission [ANSI/ASHRAE 2007].

The three counseling trailer AHUs appeared to have filters that were hand-cut from a larger piece of filter material. These filters were installed immediately behind the return air grilles into the AHUs themselves. The filter material installed in these units was not supported by any framing, but the material did seem to cover the entire return air opening to each of the AHUs. The material used was clearly made of synthetic polymers, but since the filters had no markings and appeared to be homemade, there was no way to determine the filtration efficiency of the trailer AHU filters. As mentioned previously, we could not determine which filter(s) was/were installed in the Drop Off AHU.

To prevent the spread of *M. tuberculosis,* air filters should provide a removal efficiency of greater than 90% of particles in the 1.0–3.0 μm size range (corresponding to a MERV 13 or higher). During any future HVAC design modifications, system evaluations, or retrofits, the selection of filters for use in all of the facility AHUs should be closely examined. Care should be taken when choosing more efficient filters, because increased efficiency is typically associated with increased pressure drop across the filter (resistance to air flow). Filters in the AHUs should have the highest possible efficiency (i.e., highest MERV rating) while still maintaining the air flow required for conditioning and outdoor air supply through each system.

Preventive Maintenance

With the exception of some of the window PTAC units, all of the AHUs at Community Rehabilitation Center were operational, fairly clean, and appeared to be adequately maintained. The facilities manager informed us that the ventilation filters are changed every 4–6 weeks. Unfortunately, there was no written plan outlining the preventive maintenance schedules and procedures for HVAC systems. A written HVAC operation and maintenance (O&M) plan should be developed. Currently, all preventive and emergency maintenance is managed, scheduled, and coordinated by the facilities manager, with assistance from maintenance staff. While this seems to be effective at the present time, there could be a void if the facilities manager leaves his current position or is unavailable for any significant period of time. Combining all maintenance tasks, schedules, procedures, and training requirements into a written plan would help ensure that all equipment is properly maintained at appropriate time intervals and that any emergency maintenance issues are addressed correctly. A detailed plan would also help ensure that the quality of work remains consistent as staff changes. Once developed, this written plan should be revised periodically to be current with any ventilation system and equipment modifications at the facility.

Ventilation Measurements and Indoor Air Quality

An adequate supply of outdoor air, typically delivered through the HVAC system, is necessary in any indoor environment to dilute pollutants that are released by equipment, building materials, furnishings, products, and people. In the State of Florida, the 2010 *Florida Building Code* mandates "minimum requirements to safeguard the public health, safety and general welfare through structural strength, means of egress facilities, stability, sanitation, adequate light and ventilation, energy conservation, and safety to life and property from fire and other hazards attributed to the built environment and to provide safety to fire fighters and emergency responders during emergency operations [ICC 2011]." The *Florida Building Code* applies to the "construction, alteration, movement, enlargement, replacement, repair, equipment, use and occupancy, location, maintenance, removal and demolition of every building or structure or any appurtenances connected or attached to such buildings or structures" throughout the state. The Code is based on a variety of model building codes and consensus standards from national organizations, which have been modified to fit Florida's specific needs, when necessary. When it comes to ventilation standards, in most cases, the *Florida Building Code* has adopted the recommendations published in *American National Standards Institute (ANSI)/ASHRAE Standard 62.1-2010: Ventilation for Acceptable Indoor Air Quality*. These ASHRAE recommendations provide specific details on ventilation for acceptable indoor air quality [ANSI/ASHRAE 2010a].

The 2010 *Florida Building Code* and ASHRAE 62.1-2010 recommend outdoor air supply rates that take into account people-related contaminant sources as well as building-related contaminant sources. Similarly, exhaust air flow rate requirements for some spaces are also listed. Although there are no specific guidelines for social assistance facilities, there are published guidelines applicable to Community Rehabilitation Center. These outdoor air supply and exhaust air requirements are summarized in Table 2. Table 2 also lists the default occupant densities for various spaces. These default values, given in terms of number of occupants per 1000 square feet, are provided by the *Florida Building Code* and ASHRAE to assist building and HVAC system designers when actual occupant densities are unknown. Although actual occupant densities for the occupied spaces of the facility are generally known, the default values still serve as a reference to determine whether the occupant density in a given space is higher or lower than what is considered typical.

The physical and ventilation measurements we collected are presented in Table 3. The second-to-last column of the table presents the actual occupant densities in each space. Values preceded by an asterisk (*) denote areas with occupant densities above typical values (i.e., higher than the default values presented in Table 2). High occupant densities are not solely indicative of ventilation problems. Nearly all of the offices throughout the facility show high occupant densities. Yet, most of these offices are only occupied by one person. In these cases, the occupant densities are high simply because the offices are smaller than typical office spaces. While Table 3 shows numerous office spaces with high occupant densities, none of these areas are particularly of concern, unless these same offices will be used for meeting with potentially-infectious clients. However, of particular importance are the team rooms located along the long hallway of the old portion of the main building. As shown in Table 3, these rooms were ventilated by PTAC units which do not mechanically provide outdoor air to these spaces and are not part of the centralized AHU scheme. Each of the team rooms were roughly 12 feet wide by 16 feet deep, which gives an occupiable space of approximately 190 ft². If these rooms are considered lecture classrooms (see Table 2), this floor space would allow a typical occupant density of only 12 people. Exceeding 12 people in a team room could result in an increased risk of airborne disease transmission because of the close proximity of one person to another. During our visit, team rooms 18, 19, and 20 had their dividers opened to create one large classroom. Counting the instructor, there were 41 people inside the space of 576 ft². This corresponds to an occupant density of 71 occupants per 1000 ft², compared to a typical density of only 65 occupants per 1000 ft². We were told that classes this size, and potentially larger, were fairly common in the team rooms. While the preferred approach would be to install a centralized AHU to provide sufficient outdoor air to meet actual occupancy levels in these rooms, as an interim measure, it would be prudent to limit the size of the classes to 12 people or less per team room, whenever possible. If larger classes are planned, consider using the larger dining/assembly areas because of the additional space available for clients to spread out and the increased filtration and dilution of potential infectious aerosols.

The last column in Table 3 presents the outdoor air requirements for each space, as established by the 2010 *Florida Building Code* and ASHRAE. As previously noted, none of the AHUs at Community Rehabilitation Center delivered any fresh outdoor air into the building. While AHU-3 and the AHUs in the trailers could easily be modified to bring in outdoor air, AHU-1 and AHU-2 were not installed in a way that would allow them to easily bring outdoor air into the building. Before modifying any of the AHUs to bring in outdoor air, it needs to be determined whether each individual AHU has the tempering capacity to incorporate the introduction of outdoor air. If such capacity is available, introducing outdoor air through the AHU would require some modifications and result in increased annual energy costs. However, it is important to ensure that all occupied spaces in Community Rehabilitation Center are receiving adequate amounts of fresh outdoor air to inhibit airborne disease transmission and improve indoor air quality. In addition to alleviating odors and better maintaining occupant comfort, outdoor air serves to dilute infectious aerosols, such as *M. tuberculosis* droplet nuclei.

Two common approaches could be employed by Community Rehabilitation Center to introduce outdoor air into the occupied spaces (or a combination of the two). The first approach would be to make the necessary modifications to the existing AHUs to allow them to bring in the required outdoor air. This would initially require evaluation, by a knowledgeable HVAC engineer (a reputable ventilation or engineering design contractor that is familiar with ASHRAE and CDC guidelines and recommendations), of each AHU's conditioning capacity to determine if it can handle the additional tempering and dehumidification burden introduced by the outdoor air. Assuming that such conditioning capacity exists, modifying the trailer AHUs and AHU-3 on the roof of the main building should be made easier by the fact that these units are already located outdoors. The system modifications for AHU-1 and AHU-2, servicing the newer portion of the main building, and the Drop Off AHU would require more extensive modifications since the outdoor air intakes and dampers would need to be installed into the mechanical spaces housing these AHUs. Although incorporating outdoor air into the existing AHUs may be the simpler of the two solutions and could require the least capital expense, it may cost significantly more in energy over time. In their current configurations, the AHUs are simply recirculating air that is relatively close to the desired indoor temperature and humidity conditions. After circulating through the occupied space, this air requires less conditioning to return it to the desired delivery temperature and humidity levels. Once outdoor air is mixed in with the room return air, the mixed air stream introduced to each AHU will be further from the desired indoor conditions for most of the year. Each AHU will then need to work harder to dehumidify and temper the mixed air stream.

A second common method of bringing outdoor air into the occupied spaces would be to install a dedicated outdoor air system. This would involve installing a completely new AHU with ductwork extending to all occupied spaces of the main building. This strategy could also be applied separately to the trailers and drop off building. This new AHU would be sized to provide adequate outdoor air flow for the entire main building (approximately 2000 cfm) while also providing the entire capacity to temper and dehumidify this outdoor air. The new AHU should provide tempered and dehumidified (supercooled to 45°F–50°F dew point) outdoor air to each space (or existing AHU) in quantities necessary to meet *Florida Building Code* and ASHRAE outdoor air requirements. Terminal reheating or blending of this air with air delivered by the primary AHUs may be necessary to prevent thermal discomfort from the supercooled outdoor air. Conversely, multiple smaller dedicated outdoor air systems could serve the same purpose as one large system for the entire main building. Regardless of how it is accomplished, the major advantage of the dedicated outdoor air system is that it would not require major modifications to the existing AHUs, which would simply continue to recirculate air through the spaces they serve while providing air filtration, heating and cooling. Another advantage at Community Rehabilitation Center is that the dedicated outdoor air system could be shut down during nights and weekends, when the facility is unoccupied, without impacting the operation of the existing AHUs. The dedicated outdoor air system would certainly require more capital expense and more excessive renovations for the required ductwork than the first option, but it could also provide significant energy cost savings, making it a more viable long-term solution.

A knowledgeable HVAC engineer should be consulted to discuss these and other potential options for introducing outdoor air into the shelter. Options for installing a new central HVAC system servicing the offices and team rooms currently using PTAC units should be discussed as well. A new AHU with a properly designed air distribution system would provide better air flow patterns through the spaces and improved filtration through the AHU, which would reduce the likelihood of airborne disease transmission. A new efficient central system should provide better temperature control and energy savings over the existing bank of PTAC units. The size and capacity of this new AHU would depend largely on the strategies selected to introduce outdoor air to this portion of the facility, so it is important to discuss both issues simultaneously.

During our visit, we noticed that Office 8 in the newer portion of the main building served as a medical examination room. Our measurements show (see Table 3), and ventilation fog testing confirmed, that this area was properly maintained under negative pressure compared to the corridor on the other side of the door. Thus, air from outside the exam room migrates into the room, instead of the other way around. This air flow pattern helps to keep any airborne infectious agents generated inside the room from traveling to the adjacent areas. Any areas used for medical evaluations should be maintained under negative pressure relative to the surrounding areas, and the pressure relationship should be periodically tested and confirmed with a micromanometer or visual techniques like smoke tubes or flutter strips. If it is ever determined that the exam room is under positive pressure to the corridor, then negative pressure could easily be reestablished by adjusting the ductwork so more air is exhausted from the exam room than is being supplied to it.

We also inspected and tested all of the bathroom exhaust fans during our visit. In order to control humidity and odors, bathrooms should exhaust more air than the AHU is supplying. This will maintain these areas under negative pressure. Separate exhaust fans should be used to exhaust air directly outside at least 25 feet from any air intakes. There should be no recycling or re-entrainment of return/exhaust air from the bathrooms. Exhaust fans were installed and operational in all of the bathroom areas, but the existing fans in all restrooms except the women's room off the dining area were unable to maintain the spaces under negative pressure.

For high occupancy public bathrooms, 50 cfm of exhaust per toilet/urinal is recommended. For private toilets in bathrooms intended to be occupied by only one person at a time, ASHRAE 62.1-2010 specifies that the exhaust ventilation should be 25 cfm if the exhaust fan is designed to operate continuously (the *Florida Building Code* only requires 20 cfm) or 50 cfm if the exhaust fan only operates during periods of occupancy (e.g., exhaust fan controlled by a wall switch). To help maintain negative pressure in the bathrooms, the supply air flow to the spaces could be reduced or eliminated completely, since neither the 2010 *Florida Building Code* nor ASHRAE requires supply air flow to these spaces. Even if negative pressure can be maintained by adjusting the supply air flow, the performance of the restroom exhaust fans might still need to be enhanced or the fans replaced with new ones having their exhaust rates verified for compliance with the 2010 *Florida Building Code*. Bathroom fans should be operational whenever the rooms are occupied. [Note: The kitchen hood exhaust system was not evaluated at the time of the NIOSH site visit due to ongoing meal preparation activities, so it is not discussed in this report.]

While not a major concern from an airborne disease transmission standpoint, temperature and relative humidity (RH) affect the perception of comfort in an indoor environment. The perception of thermal comfort is related to one's metabolic heat production, the transfer of heat to the environment, physiological adjustments, and body temperature. Heat transfer from the body to the environment is influenced by factors such as temperature, humidity, air movement, personal activities, and clothing. *ANSI/ASHRAE Standard 55-2010: Thermal Environmental Conditions for Human Occupancy* specifies conditions in which 80% or more of the occupants are expected to find the environment thermally acceptable [ANSI/ASHRAE 2010b]. Assuming slow air movement and 50% RH, the operative temperatures recommended by ASHRAE range from 68.5°F–76°F in the winter, and from 75.5°F–80.5°F in the summer (see Table 4). The difference between the two temperature ranges is largely due to seasonal clothing selection. ASHRAE also recommends that RH be maintained at or below 65%. The U.S. Environmental Protection Agency recommends maintaining indoor relative humidity between 30–50% because excessive humidity can promote the growth of microorganisms [EPA 2012]. Temperature and RH levels were not recorded during our visit. Regardless, we recommend maintaining the indoor temperature and RH levels within the ranges established by ASHRAE to provide the most comfortable environment to clients at Community Rehabilitation Center. Consistently meeting the 30–50% RH recommendation would be significantly easier if a dedicated outdoor air system is installed to introduce conditioned outdoor air to the facility, as explained above.

Respiratory Protection

During an outbreak of airborne infectious disease, there could be instances when staff members find themselves in close contact with guests suspected of being infectious. One example would be a van driver transporting clients to/from Community Rehabilitation Center. Ideally, these cases would be identified during the administrative screening process. When these circumstances cannot be avoided, it is wise to consider the availability of respiratory protection to protect staff members. The first step toward the implementation of respirator use is to develop a document that clearly outlines a formal respiratory protection program. The Occupational Safety and Health Administration (OSHA) Respiratory Protection standard (29 Code of Federal Regulations [CFR] 1910.134) outlines the requirements for comprehensive respiratory protection programs. In accordance with 29 CFR 1910.134, a written Respiratory Protection Program, with an identified program administrator, is required for any facility that requires employees to wear respirators. The program must include training, medical evaluations, and respirators at no cost to employees or staff required to wear respirators on the job. Initial fit testing by a trained individual is required for all employees that will potentially wear a respirator. Annual fit testing is required after that, with additional fit testing upon major changes to the facial features of the respirator user (i.e. major weight gain/loss, change in facial hair, scarring, etc.).

To comply with applicable OSHA regulations regarding respiratory protection, we recommend that Community Rehabilitation Center create a written respiratory protection program as outlined in 29 CFR 1910.134, appoint a program administrator, and initiate training and initial fit testing for employees. Many online resources exist to assist in the development of a respiratory protection program. OSHA has published a Respiratory Protection informational booklet online (http://www.osha.gov/Publications/OSHA3079/osha3079.html) and a more detailed Small Entity Compliance Guide for the Revised Respiratory Protection Standard (http://www.osha.gov/Publications/3384small-entity-for-respiratory-protection-standard-rev.pdf) to explain all parts of an appropriate respiratory protection program and how to comply. The Small Entity Compliance Guide also contains a sample respiratory protection program in Attachment 4 that can be used as a model program. The Washington State Department of Labor and Industries has also developed a user-friendly, fillable template that is helpful in developing a respiratory protection program at http://www.lni.wa.gov/Safety/Basics/Programs/Accident/Samples/RespProtectguide2.doc.

The DCHD, Florida Department of Health, local healthcare facilities or fire/ambulance stations can potentially assist with training and fit testing the employees required to wear respirators. Alternatively, qualitative fit testing kits (Bitrix™) can be purchased for around $200.00. When paired with a trained and competent fit test administrator (see 29 CFR 1910.134), these kits would allow cost-effective, on-site fit testing annually.

Conclusions

Since the increase in cases of TB disease in 2010, Community Rehabilitation Center has taken significant steps to improve the administrative controls at the facility. Important lines of communication between the facility and DCHD have been established, and improvements to staff training and awareness of TB symptoms have been made. Helping to identify clients displaying symptoms of TB disease or those listed on the DCHD target screening lists will help further reduce the potential for future cases of TB disease and bring the ongoing outbreak under control. Having consistent protective strategies upon suspect case identification is also important. While enhanced administrative controls are now in place, there is no written ICP established at the facility, and Community Rehabilitation Center administrators are encouraged to promptly coordinate with DCHD and the Florida Department of Health to establish one.

From an environmental control perspective, the three central AHUs installed in the main building and the AHUs in both trailers were well maintained and appeared to be functioning properly. The Drop Off AHU seemed to function properly, but we were unable to visually inspect the unit during our visit. Filters with a MERV 8 efficiency value are used in all of the main building AHUs, and the filters were reportedly changed every 6 weeks. Filtration efficiency for the trailer AHUs could not be determined. The spaces down the longest hallway in the old portion of the main building were ventilated with under-window PTAC units, and some of the units were not functional during our visit. The preventive maintenance program in place is managed by the current facilities manager. Aside from issues with some of the PTAC units, the program seems to be effective although it had not been formalized into a written preventive maintenance or O&M plan for the facility AHUs.

None of the AHUs at Community Rehabilitation Center were providing fresh outdoor air to the occupied spaces, as required by the 2010 *Florida Building Code* and ASHRAE guidelines. Given the number of clients served by the facility and the close proximity of clients to one another in some of the occupied spaces, it is important that these spaces are receiving adequate amounts of outdoor air. In addition to alleviating odors and better maintaining occupant comfort, outdoor air serves to dilute infectious aerosols, such as *M. tuberculosis* droplet nuclei responsible for TB transmission. With some simple adjustments to AHU-3 and all three trailer AHUs, and with more extensive modifications to AHU-1, AHU-2, and the Drop Off AHU, the existing equipment might be made to provide the necessary outdoor air. Another alternative would be to augment the existing AHUs with the installation of new dedicated outdoor air systems to provide outdoor air. A knowledgeable HVAC engineer should be consulted to discuss options for introducing outdoor air to the shelter. During those discussions, options for replacing the PTAC units in the old portion of the main building with a new, efficient central AHU should be investigated. Once these changes have been implemented, other ventilation equipment and/or supplemental ultraviolet germicidal irradiation systems could be investigated if additional environmental controls are desired.

For instances where improvements to administrative and environmental controls do not sufficiently mitigate the risk for disease transmission, respiratory protection might be necessary. There was no formal respiratory protection program in place during our visit, but such a program should be implemented at the facility. Having this program in place will provide additional protection to Community Rehabilitation Center staff working in close proximity to clients with suspected TB or other airborne diseases. Any respirator use at the facility should be covered by an OSHA-mandated respiratory protection program.

Administratively, a positive approach is being taken toward reducing the likelihood of future TB transmission at Community Rehabilitation Center. However, the ventilation systems clearly need some attention to further reduce the risk. While ventilation systems and other environmental control systems cannot guarantee prevention of future TB disease transmission, improving the environmental controls will reduce the potential for airborne disease transmission, along with providing better indoor air quality throughout the facility. The following recommendations are aimed at improving the overall infection control program at Community Rehabilitation Center, with specific emphasis on improvements to the existing environmental controls so they meet all applicable standards and guidelines.

Recommendations

Based on our assessment of environmental controls at Community Rehabilitation Center, we have developed the following list of recommendations, in order of priority:

1. **Continue to improve and enhance the TB administrative controls at the facility and develop a written Infection Control Plan.**

   - Continue working with the DCHD to screen facility staff and guests for TB disease.

   - With input from DCHD, develop specific procedures for handling a suspected or confirmed case of TB disease.

   - Continue educating facility staff on the signs and symptoms of TB disease so they can readily identify suspect cases and implement established precautions.

   - Consider displaying informational posters about TB signs and symptoms to educate clients.

   - Consider displaying signs encouraging proper cough etiquette and hand hygiene.

   - Develop a formal written TB Infection Control Plan. Seek guidance and input from DCHD and the Florida Department of Health. The plan should include:

   o All aspects of the TB infection control program and associated responsibilities, especially those functions requiring coordination with other agencies, such as the local and state health departments

   o The improved administrative controls put in place at Community Rehabilitation Center since the beginning of the TB outbreak

   o Input from ventilation staff. Obtaining input from ventilation maintenance staff serves to strengthen the environmental control section of the plan while giving maintenance staff additional insight into the ventilation requirements for reducing or preventing airborne disease transmission.

   o Schedule for updating and revising the ICP

2. **Introduce the required amounts of fresh outdoor air to all occupied spaces.**

- There are multiple options that can allow adequate outdoor air to be supplied to the facility. All options, including the associated capital, maintenance, and annual operating costs should be considered. Work with a reputable ventilation or engineering contractor familiar with the current *Florida Building Code*, ASHRAE, and CDC guidelines to select the best option for Community Rehabilitation Center.

- Install a new, efficient central AHU to replace all existing PTAC units used in spaces down the longest hallway of the older portion of the main building. Sizing and selection of this new AHU should be done at the same time decisions are made on the best method to introduce outdoor air into the facility.

3. **Improve filtration efficiency in all AHUs.** Select higher efficiency filters (higher MERV ratings) for use in each AHU, as long as the new filters do not adversely impact the required air flow delivery capacity of the AHUs.

4. **Develop and implement an OSHA respiratory protection program in accordance with 29 CFR 1910.134.** To meet the OSHA requirements, you must:

- Designate a program administrator who is qualified by appropriate training or experience to administer or oversee the program and conduct the required program evaluations

- Provide respirators, training, and medical evaluations at no cost to employees required to wear respirators on the job

- Develop a written program with worksite-specific procedures when respirators are necessary or required by the employer. The written respiratory protection program needs to include:

- Respirator types and proper respirator selection
- Required medical evaluations for employees prior to respirator use
- Procedures for initial and annual respirator fit testing
- Instructions for proper respirator use
- Information on appropriate respirator maintenance and care
- Initial and yearly training requirements for respirator users
- Procedures for evaluating the effectiveness of the respiratory protection program

- Update the respiratory protection program as necessary to reflect changes in workplace conditions that affect respirator use.

5. **Ensure all bathrooms are maintained under negative pressure and exhaust fans meet required performance specifications.** Bathrooms currently under positive pressure could be brought under negative pressure by reducing or eliminating the supply air flow to the spaces. Even if negative pressure can be maintained by adjusting the supply air flow, the performance of the bathroom exhaust should still comply with the 2010 *Florida Building Code* and ASHRAE requirements. Ensure that all exhaust air from bathrooms is exhausted directly outside and that no return air from bathrooms is recirculated back to an AHU or entrained in the outdoor air entering any current or future AHU.

6. **After all of the ventilation systems are updated and functioning properly, develop a comprehensive, written HVAC O&M plan.** The O&M Plan should include:

- Preventive maintenance schedules and all regularly scheduled maintenance tasks (filter changes, fan belt inspections, etc.) and identify personnel who is responsible for conducting each task
- Written procedures for each maintenance task to ensure the work is done properly each time, regardless of who performs the work
- Training requirements for maintenance staff
- A method for logging maintenance activities for each AHU
- A method for updating or revising the O&M Plan as procedures or systems change

Outline of Future NIOSH Involvement

This report will serve to close out NIOSH Technical Assistance at Community Rehabilitation Center. However, we understand that the work outlined in the recommendations above will take several months to complete and will represent a significant investment of time and financial resources. As the work proceeds, NIOSH could assist by:

- Reviewing any Requests for Proposal developed to initiate the bidding process
- Reviewing any bids received in response to Requests for Proposals for technical content
- Providing technical assistance related to any environmental control strategies

It is not necessary for NIOSH to be on-site during any ventilation renovations. Yet, as projects are initiated, we can assist you by reviewing:

- Proposed modification strategies for outdoor air introduction
- Preliminary design schematics or equipment selection documents
- Air flow testing and balancing reports
- Final project documents, including as-built drawings, sequences of operations, and proper equipment set points

Once the renovations are complete, if additional NIOSH assistance is desired or warranted, the request for technical assistance can be reopened.

References

ANSI/ASHRAE (American National Standards Institute/American Society of Heating, Ventilating and Air-Conditioning Engineers) [2007]. Method of testing general ventilation air-cleaning devices for removal efficiency by particle size. Atlanta, GA: American Society of Heating, Refrigerating and Air-Conditioning Engineers. Standard 52.2-2007.

ANSI/ASHRAE [2010a]. Ventilation for acceptable indoor air quality. Atlanta, GA: American Society of Heating, Refrigerating and Air-Conditioning Engineers. Standard 62.1-2010.

ANSI/ASHRAE [2010b]. Thermal environmental conditions for human occupancy. Atlanta, GA: American Society of Heating, Refrigerating and Air-Conditioning Engineers. Standard 55-2010.

Barry MA, Wall C, Shirley L, Bernardo J, Schwingl P, Brigandi E, Lamb GA [1986]. Tuberculosis screening in Boston's homeless shelters. Public Health Rep 101(5):487-498.

CDC (Centers for Disease Control and Prevention) [1985]. Drug-resistant tuberculosis among the homeless—Boston. MMWR 34:429-431.

CDC [1992]. Prevention and control of tuberculosis among homeless persons (ACET). MMWR 41(RR-5):001.

CDC [2003a]. Tuberculosis outbreak in a homeless population—Portland, Maine, 2002-2003. MMWR 52(48):1184-1185.

CDC [2003b]. TB outbreak among homeless persons—King County, Washington, 2002-2003. MMWR 52(49):1209-1210.

CDC [2005a]. Tuberculosis transmission in a homeless shelter population—New York, 2000-2003. MMWR 54(06):149-152.

CDC [2005b]. Guidelines for preventing the transmission of *Mycobacterium tuberculosis* in health-care settings, 2005. MMWR 54(RR-17):1-141.

CDC [2006]. Prevention and control of tuberculosis in correctional and detention facilities: Recommendations from CDC. MMWR 55(RR-9):1-54.

EPA (US Environmental Protection Agency) [2012]. The inside story: A guide to indoor air quality http://www.epa.gov/iaq/pubs/insidestory.html. Date accessed: February 22, 2013.

ICC (International Code Council, Inc.) [2011]. *Florida building code* 2010: Mechanical (chapter 4, ventilation). Country Club Hills, IL: International Code Council, Inc.

Knopf SA [1914]. Tuberculosis as a cause and result of poverty. J Am Med Assoc 63(20):1720-1725.

McAdam JM, Brickner PW, Scharer LL, Crocco JA, Duff AE [1990]. The spectrum of tuber-culosis in a New York City men's shelter clinic (1982-1988). Chest 97:798-805.

Nolan CM, Elarth AM, Barr H, Saeed AM, Risser DR [1991]. An outbreak of tuberculosis in a shelter for homeless men: A description of its evolution and control. Am Rev Respir Dis 143:257-261.

Slutkin G [1986]. Management of tuberculosis in urban homeless indigents. Public Health Rep 101(5):481-485.

Table 1. General air-handling unit (AHU) information

NIOSH AHU Identifier	Physical Location of AHU	Main Locations Served by AHU[A]	AHU Manufacturer[B]	AHU Model Number[B]	Proper Filter Configuration in AHU[C,D]	Actual Filter Configuration in AHU[B,D]
AHU-1	Main Building – New Section, Mechanical Room Adjacent to Office 14	All Offices and Hallways of Main Building – New Section	Ruud	RHGF-100ZK949	(4) 16 × 25 × 1	(4) 16 × 25 × 1
AHU-2	Main Building, New Section, Mechanical Room Adjacent to Office 14	Dining/Activity Areas of Main Building – New Section	Ruud	RHGE-150ZK949	(6) 20 × 25 × 1	(6) 20 × 25 × 1
AHU-3	Rooftop of Main Building – Old Section	Area 3, Offices 4-11, and Copier Room 12 of Main Building – Old Section	Carrier	50TCQD12A-2B5A0A0A0	(4) 20 × 20 × 2 (RA) & (1) 20 × 24 × 1 (OA)[E]	(4) 20 × 20 × 2 (RA) & (1) 20 × 24 × 1 (OA)[E]
Drop Off AHU	Attic Space of Drop Off Building	All Drop Off Building	Unknown[F]	Unknown[F]	Unknown[F]	Unknown[F]
Small Trailer AHU	North End of Small Trailer	All of Trailer 1	Unknown[G]	Unknown[G]	Unknown[G]	Homemade[H]
Large Trailer AHUs[I]	South End of Large Trailer	All of Trailer 2	Eubank Manufacturing Enterprises, Inc.	W36CF10B1F00A	Unknown[G]	Homemade[H]

[A] May not represent all locations served by the AHU
[B] Information collected during visual inspection of AHU
[C] Information gathered from product data specific to each AHU model published by respective AHU manufacturer
[D] Value in parenthesis represents the number of filters, dimensions are width × height × depth in units of inches
[E] RA = Return Air; OA = Outdoor Air (outdoor air damper was completely closed on this AHU)
[F] Ventilation measurements were taken in the area supplied by the Drop Off AHU, but access to the AHU was not readily available during the NIOSH visit.
[G] Labels and stickers on the Small Trailer AHU were missing or faded so they could not be read.
[H] Rough, hand-cut, homemade filters were installed in the Small Trailer AHU and both Large Trailer AHUs.
[I] The Large Trailer had two identical AHUs, both on the south end of the trailer.

Table 2. Applicable outdoor air supply flow rates, minimum exhaust air flow rates, and default occupancy densities from the 2010 Florida Building Code and ASHRAE Standard 62.1-2010[A]

Occupancy Category	People Outdoor Air Flow Rate (cfm/person)[B]	Area Outdoor Air Flow Rate (cfm/ft²)[C]	Minimum Exhaust Air Flow Rate[D]	Default Occupant Density (#/1000 ft²)[E]
Office Spaces	5	0.06	—	5
Conference Rooms	5	0.06	—	50
Multipurpose Assembly Spaces	5	0.06	—	120
Reception Areas	5	0.06	—	30
Break Rooms[F]	5[F]	0.12[F]	—	50[F]
Occupiable Dry Storage Rooms[F]	5[F]	0.06[F]	—	2[F]
Occupiable Liquid/Gel Storage Rooms[F]	5[F]	0.12[F]	—	2[F]
Unoccupiable Storage Rooms[G]	—	0.12[G]	—	—
Lobbies/Prefunction Spaces	7.5	0.06	—	30
Lecture Classrooms	7.5	0.06	—	65
Computer Labs	10	0.12	—	25
Dining Rooms	7.5	0.18	—	70
Central Kitchens	7.5[F]	0.12[F]	0.7 cfm/ft²[C]	70
Public Bathrooms	—	—	50 or 70 cfm/toilet and/or urinal[H]	—
Private Bathrooms	—	—	25 or 50 cfm[I]	—

[A] Requirements published in: *2010 Florida Building Code: Mechanical* (Chapter 4, Ventilation). International Code Council, Inc., Country Club Hills, IL (2011) and American National Standards Institute (ANSI)/American Society of Heating, Refrigerating and Air-Conditioning Engineers (ASHRAE). *Ventilation for Acceptable Indoor Air Quality, Standard 62.1-2010*. ASHRAE, Atlanta, GA (2010). In nearly all cases, the *2010 Florida Building Code* has adopted ventilation recommendations directly from ASHRAE Standard 62.1-2010.
[B] cfm/person = cubic feet per minute (also commonly shown as ft³/min) per person typically in the occupied space
[C] cfm/ft² = cubic feet per minute (also commonly shown as ft³/min) per square feet of occupied space
[D] Mechanical exhaust should be released directly outdoors at least 25 feet away from air intakes. Recirculation of exhaust air back into the building should be avoided.
[E] #/1000ft² = number of people per 1000 square feet of occupied space. These values are typical occupant densities in spaces that are useful for building/HVAC system design. If actual occupant densities are known, they should be used instead of these default values.
[F] Requirements are only published in ASHRAE Standard 62.1-2010. No directly corresponding values appear in the *2010 Florida Building Code*.
[G] Requirements are only published in the *2010 Florida Building Code*. No directly corresponding values appear in ASHRAE Standard 62.1-2010.
[H] Provide the higher rate when periods of heavy use are expected to occur (e.g. prior to guests leaving in the morning). If periods of heavy use are not anticipated, the lower rate may be used.
[I] These rates are for bathrooms intended for use by one person at a time. If exhaust fans are operated continuously, the lower rate may be used. If exhaust fans are operated intermittently (e.g., fans activated by a light switch), the higher rate should be used.

Table 3. Ventilation observations, occupant densities, and recommended outdoor air flow for areas served by central AHUs or where guests congregate

Space[A]	AHU Serving Space	Return Flow from Space (cfm)[B]	Supply Flow into Space (cfm)[B]	Approximate Area of Space (ft²)[C]	Typical Occupants in Space[D]	Occupant Density (#/1000 ft²)[D,E,F]	Recommended Outdoor Air Flow (cfm)[B,G]
Main Building – New Section							
Reception	AHU-1	170	360	315	1	3	23.9
Conference Room	AHU-1	140	85	205	6	29	42.3
Office 1	AHU-1	0	80	110	1	*9	11.6
Office 2	AHU-1	85	50	110	1	*9	11.6
Office 3	AHU-1	75	70	110	1	*9	11.6
Office 4	AHU-1	85	85	110	1	*9	11.6
Office 5	AHU-1	80	0	110	1	*9	11.6
Office 6	AHU-1	110	120	185	1	5	16.1
Office 7	AHU-1	90	110	245	1	4	19.7
Office 8 (Medical)[H]	AHU-1	130[H]	90[H]	170	2	*12	20.2
Office 9	AHU-1	70	80	125	2	*16	17.5
Office 10	AHU-1	65	65	130	1	*8	12.8
Office 11	AHU-1	90	80	130	1	*8	12.8
Office 12	AHU-1	70	90	145	1	*7	13.7
Office 13	AHU-1	None[I]	140	160	1	*6	14.6
Men's Room (Just Outside Dining Area)	AHU-1	145[J]	150	220	N/A[K]	N/A[K]	N/A[K]
Office 14 (Executive Director)	AHU-1	210	110	200	1	5	17.0
Network/IT Administration	AHU-1	90[J]	55	105	1	10	11.3
Restroom Adjacent to Office 14	AHU-1	40[J]	70	55	N/A[K]	N/A[K]	N/A[K]
Dining/Activity Area (NE Half, Off Hallway 1)	AHU-2	1670	1410	1440	60	42	386.4/709.2[L]
Dining/Activity Area (SW Half, Off Hallway 2)	AHU-2	1550	1315	1650	60	36	399.0/747.0[L]
Women's Room (Inside Dining Area)	AHU-2	200[J]	155	220	N/A[K]	N/A[K]	N/A[K]
Kitchen	AHU-2	None[J,M]	905	375	4	11	75

Table 3 (continued). Ventilation observations, occupant densities, and recommended outdoor air flow for areas served by central AHUs or where guests congregate

Space[A]	AHU Serving Space	Return Flow from Space (cfm)[B]	Supply Flow into Space (cfm)[B]	Approximate Area of Space (ft²)[C]	Typical Occupants in Space[D]	Occupant Density (#/1000 ft²)[D,E,F]	Recommended Outdoor Air Flow (cfm)[B,G]
Main Building – Old Section							
Area 3	AHU-3	CNM[N]	170	280	0	0	33.6
Office 4	AHU-3	CNM[N]	190	120	1	*8	12.2
Office 5	AHU-3	CNM[N]	200	130	1	*8	12.8
Office 6	AHU-3	CNM[N]	190	115	1	*9	11.9
Office 7	AHU-3	CNM[N]	270	120	1	*8	12.2
Office 8	AHU-3	CNM[N]	200	105	1	*10	11.3
Office 9	AHU-3	CNM[N]	Obs[O]	375	1	3	27.5
Office 10	AHU-3	CNM[N]	Obs[O]	160	1	*6	14.6
Office 11	AHU-3	CNM[N]	180	135	1	*7	13.1
Copier Room 12	AHU-3	CNM[N]	300	230	1	4	18.8
Unnumbered Office Off Copier Room 12	AHU-3	145[P]	90	185	1	5	16.1
Office 13	AHU-3	CNM[N]	160	155	1	*6	14.3
Team Room 18	PTAC[Q]	---[Q]	---[Q]	190	15	*79	86.4
Team Room 19	PTAC[Q]	---[Q]	---[Q]	190	15	*79	86.4
Team Room 20	PTAC[Q]	---[Q]	---[Q]	190	15	*79	86.4
Team Room 21	PTAC[Q]	---[Q]	---[Q]	190	15	*79	86.4
Team Room 22	PTAC[Q]	---[Q]	---[Q]	190	15	*79	86.4
Team Room 23	PTAC[Q]	---[Q]	---[Q]	190	15	*79	86.4
Team Room 24	PTAC[Q]	---[Q]	---[Q]	190	15	*79	86.4

Table 3 (continued). Ventilation observations, occupant densities, and recommended outdoor air flow for areas served by central AHUs or where guests congregate

Space[A]	AHU Serving Space	Return Flow from Space (cfm)[B]	Supply Flow into Space (cfm)[B]	Approximate Area of Space (ft²)[C]	Typical Occupants in Space[D]	Occupant Density (#/1000 ft²)[D,E,F]	Recommended Outdoor Air Flow (cfm)[B,G]
Drop-Off Building							
Game/Activity Area	Drop Off AHU	415	370	485	30	62	179.1
Small Trailer							
Adult Basic Education Area	Small Trailer AHU	145	210	335	4	12	40.1
Storage Room	Small Trailer AHU	70	305	130	0	0	15.6
Office Area	Small Trailer AHU	40	360	130	1	*8	12.8
Large Trailer							
Office 1	Large Trailer AHUs	Wall[R]	160	115	1	*9	11.9
Office 2	Large Trailer AHUs	Wall[R]	110	115	1	*9	11.9
Waiting Area	Large Trailer AHUs	None[J]	70	185	1	5	16.1
Office 3	Large Trailer AHUs	Wall[R]	80	90	1	*11	10.4
Office 4	Large Trailer AHUs	Wall[R]	60	85	1	*12	10.1
Office 5	Large Trailer AHUs	Wall[R]	95	110	1	*9	11.6
Restroom	Large Trailer AHUs	30[J]	115	65	N/A[K]	N/A[K]	N/A[K]
Office 6	Large Trailer AHUs	Wall[R]	100	95	1	*11	10.7
Back Reception Area	Large Trailer AHUs	Wall[R]	40	130	1	*8	12.8

[A] May not represent all locations served by the AHU
[B] cfm = cubic feet per minute (also commonly shown as ft³/min)
[C] ft² = square feet
[D] Occupant numbers estimated by visual observation during NIOSH visit
[E] #/1000 ft² = number of occupants per 1000 ft² of occupied floor space. Calculated by dividing the number of typical occupants in the space by the approximate area of the space and multiplying by 1000
[F] Entries preceded by an asterisk (*) represent spaces where the actual occupant density likely exceeds the default occupant density presented in Table 2.
[G] Calculated based on recommendations published in: American National Standards Institute (ANSI)/American Society of Heating, Refrigerating and Air-Conditioning Engineers (ASHRAE). Ventilation for Acceptable Indoor Air Quality, Standard 62.1-2010. ASHRAE, Atlanta, GA (2010) and the 2010 Florida Building Code: Mechanical (Chapter 4, Ventilation). International Code Council, Inc., Country Club Hills, IL (2011). In nearly all cases, the 2010 Florida Building Code has adopted ventilation recommendations directly from ASHRAE Standard 62.1-2010.

H Areas where medical examinations and/or procedures are performed should be maintained under negative pressure compared to adjacent areas (i.e., more air should be exhausted from the space than is supplied to the space). This space was under negative pressure during the NIOSH visit.

I There was/were no return grille(s) in this space. Only supply vent(s) was/were present.

J This area was equipped with a switch activated exhaust fan designed for intermittent use when the space is occupied.

K N/A = not applicable. Neither ASHRAE Standard 62.1-2010 nor the 2010 Florida Building Code include outdoor air recommendations for restrooms and bathrooms. Instead, for public bathrooms, the recommendation is 50 cfm of exhaust from the space per toilet or urinal when periods of heavy use are not expected. Bathroom exhaust may be made up entirely of transfer air from adjacent spaces (i.e., no direct supply air to the space is required) and only a maximum of 10% of the exhaust air is permitted to be recycled.

L ASHRAE Standard 62.1-2010 and the 2010 Florida Building Code: Mechanical (Chapter 4, Ventilation) provide separate outdoor air recommendations for assembly spaces and dining rooms. Both numbers are reported here (assembly space/dining area).

M Does not include air pulled from the area by kitchen exhaust hoods. Air flow measurements through exhaust hoods were not taken.

N CNM = could not measure. Return air passed around light fixtures into the plenum space above the drop ceiling. Measurements of the return air could not be taken accurately during the NIOSH visit.

O Obs = obstructed. Air flow measurements could not be taken because the supply vents were obstructed by furniture, storage boxes, shelves, etc.

P This was an unducted return grille through the drop ceiling into the ceiling plenum.

Q These areas were ventilated by packaged terminal air conditioner (PTAC) units that did not provide outdoor air to the spaces and are not part of the central ventilation system. No supply or return measurements were taken.

R Return air from these spaces flowed through grilles in the walls into other occupied spaces until finally returning to the AHUs on the end of the trailer. No measurements of this return air were taken.

Table 4. ASHRAE indoor relative humidity and temperature recommendations[A]

Relative Humidity	Winter Temperatures[B]	Summer Temperatures[B]
30%[C]	69.5°F to 77.0°F	75.5°F to 81.5°F
40%	69.0°F to 76.5°F	75.5°F to 81.0°F
50%[D]	68.5°F to 76.0°F	75.0°F to 80.5°F

[A] Adapted from: ANSI/ASHRAE. Thermal Environmental Conditions for Human Occupancy, Standard 55-2010. American Society of Heating, Refrigerating and Air-Conditioning Engineers, Atlanta, GA. (2010)
[B] Applies to occupants wearing typical summer and winter clothing, with a sedentary to light activity level
[C] Humidity levels below 30% may cause irritated mucus membranes, dry eyes, and sinus discomfort.
[D] The U.S. Environmental Protection Agency recommends maintaining indoor relative humidity below 60% and ideally in a range from 30% to 50% to prevent mold growth.

The Health Hazard Evaluation Program investigates possible health hazards in the workplace under the authority of Section 20(a)(6) of the Occupational Safety and Health Act of 1970, 29 U.S.C. 669(a)(6). The Health Hazard Evaluation Program also provides, upon request, technical assistance to federal, state, and local agencies to control occupational health hazards and to prevent occupational illness and disease. Regulations guiding the Program can be found in Title 42, Code of Federal Regulations, Part 85; Requests for Health Hazard Evaluations (42 CFR 85).

Acknowledgments

This report was prepared by Stephen B. Martin, Jr., R. Brent Lawrence, and Michael C. Beaty of the Field Studies Branch (FSB), Division of Respiratory Disease Studies (DRDS) and Kenneth R. Mead of the Engineering and Physical Hazards Branch, Division of Applied Research and Technology. Desktop publishing was performed by Tia McClelland (FSB/ DRDS).

Availability of Report

Copies of this report have been sent to representatives from Community Rehabilitation Center, DCHD, the Florida Department of Health, CDC/NCHHSTP/DTBE, and the OSHA Regional Office. This report is not copyrighted and may be freely reproduced.

This report is available at http://www.cdc.gov/niosh/hhe/reports/pdfs/2012-0263-3181.pdf.

Recommended citation for this report:
NIOSH [2013]. Health hazard evaluation report: Evaluation of environmental controls at social assistance facility (Community Rehabilitation Center) associated with a tuberculosis outbreak – Florida. By Martin, Jr. SB, Mead KR, Lawrence RB, Beaty MC. Morgantown, WV: U.S. Department of Health and Human Services, Centers for Disease Control and Prevention, National Institute for Occupational Safety and Health, NIOSH Report No. 2012-0263-3181.